NATURAL DECEPTION

A Sobering Look at the Truth Behind the Organic Food Industry

By Joey Lott

www.joeylotthealth.com

Publishing services provided by 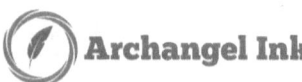 Archangel Ink

ISBN: 151866606X
ISBN-13: 978-1518666063

Table of Contents

4

What Led to This

I grew up smack dab in the middle of the American Midwest in the 1980s—a place and time in which the term "organic" might as well have been Greek and "natural" meant a cornfield (as opposed to a parking lot). When I was ten years old, I sported a mullet, and for a pastime I would ride my bicycle a mile to the Tastee Treet to eat a cup of soft-serve ice cream with M&Ms mixed into it, buy a pack of baseball cards, and chew the pink stick of gum that came with the cards on the ride home. I had no idea that any other way existed; that was what *everyone* did as far as I knew.

When I was nineteen years old, I left college and took a Greyhound bus to Los Angeles, California, to "find my fortune." Initially I was making just $250 a week, so price was one of the biggest considerations when it came to food. Purchasing produce from the farmers market afforded me the best price *and* the best quality, and it was through my weekly trips to the farmers market in Hollywood that I began to discover the differences in farming practices among the many vendors.

As my income allowed and my education increased, I began to buy an increasing amount of food that was described as "organic." Initially, organic standards in California were set by the California Certified Organic Farmers (CCOF) organization, and many of the vendors at the market were certified by CCOF. But by the early 2000s, the U.S. Department of Agriculture (USDA) took over, making CCOF a certifying agency enforcing the standards of the USDA. When that happened, I recall many vendors bemoaning the "death of organic," claiming that the USDA standards were "too lax." Furthermore, many of the farmers who had previously displayed CCOF signs stopped doing so; though no one ever said so explicitly, I got the impression that the costs of certification increased substantially.

Still, I was young, I was urban, and though I was at the time a raving liberal, I didn't care enough to peer too deeply beneath the surface. I was sold on the idea of organic and natural as the moral high ground and the potential savior of all life on the planet. So when I moved to Boston a few years later, a virtual food wasteland compared to California, I shopped exclusively at Whole Foods Market, buying only certified organic foods. It wasn't until I moved to a smaller town a few years later that I began to question my loyalty.

I purchased a 25-pound bag of beans (I ate a lot of beans in my vegan days) in 2008, and for the first time, I noticed the *source* of the food. In that case, I noticed that the beans, though certified organic (by the USDA), had been grown in China. *How*, I wondered, *could beans grown in China be certified organic by the USDA?* And that began my deepening curiosity into the matter.

Subsequently, I developed an increasing interest in getting "closer" to my food. I strived to produce as much of my own food as possible, which at most has been 2 percent, so I'm no Joel Salatin or Eliot Coleman. I moved to rural locations and began volunteering on organic farms. I started gardening. I helped neighbors who kept livestock. And what I found was that it was *really* hard to produce food according to my own strict standards of healthfulness and purity. Not only was it really hard, but almost *no one* was doing it—not on a small scale and most certainly not on a large scale.

Admittedly, my standards were unnecessarily rigid and obsessive—in a word: unreasonable. But this process began to open my eyes to a reality that I had been blinded to by my own membership in the church of organic for all those years: the organic and natural food industry has painted an idealized picture that we are meant to believe while the truth is quite different.

What I have come to find is that organic and natural is a big business. And, not surprisingly, big business is now in the business of organic and natural. The *story* of organic is a nice one—small, diversified farms that are family-owned and operated and on which the land and animals are treated with respect and kindness. We're meant to believe that organic food production is a revolution that can transform human relationships with the land and with animals into something wholly sustainable. In fact, depending on one's inclinations, the organic story might even border on the religious. But my experiences have suggested to me that the truth of *most* certified organic food production—at least in the United States, which is the focus on my investigation—is not as we've been led to believe.

This book is intended to explore the question, *is organic food production really better for our bodies, the animals in the system, or our world?* Yes, it is true that small-scale, local, family-owned-and-operated organic farms do exist. But the truth is that the overwhelming majority of organic food production is happening on an industrial scale. So in this book, I want to look specifically at large-scale organic food like Cal-Organics, Earthbound Farms, Cascadian Farms, Organic Valley, Horizon, and their ilk. We pay a great deal more for organic, explaining why Whole Foods Market has the nickname Whole Paycheck, but what are we paying for? Are we paying for healthier food? Are we paying for better conditions and treatment for animals? Are we paying for a healthier world? And is organic actually delivering value for our money? Or is it just lining the corporate coffers?

Let's find out.

The Plight of Small and Local

It seems likely that for the overwhelming majority of history on Earth, the emphasis of all systems and economies has been local. Sure, in a larger context, everything is interconnected, but up until the last few hundred years the leverage has been applied and felt *locally*. In other words, until very recently, food was generally sourced from only as far away as one could walk or float; North Americans had never seen cinnamon or broccoli or wheat, and Africans had never tasted tomatoes or bison.

I don't have to tell you, of course, that things are different today. I can get in a car and drive thirty minutes to a store in which I can find Atlantic salmon, Argentinian apples, oranges from California, bananas from Ecuador, pumpkin seeds from China, Italian tomato sauce, and Hawaiian-grown ginger root—all despite the fact that I live in the desert at 6000 feet above sea level. And I'm not alone. This is true of just about everyone in the United States.

These foods are part of a massive food production and distribution system. For the most part, that is true regardless of whether the food is certified organic or not. True, there are still small food producers, and the interest in local food seems to have increased in recent years. However, what is not clear is whether the growth of interest in local food is outpacing the ravenous appetite for certified organic. And, as we'll see in this book, the corporate interests involved in organic certification are at odds with local food production.

When I was a child, I lived across the street from what was then a small family farm. My father had worked on the farm when he was a teenager, and his sister had married one of the farmer's sons. I played in the fields with my cousin and the youngest of the farmer's sons, who was only a year older than me. We went fishing in the pond behind the barns.

The farm wasn't an idyllic one by purist standards. The farmer sprayed synthetic pesticides on the crops and planted acres of monocrops. I recall the stench of what smelled like a mix of rotting eggs and cabbage as the sulfurous pesticide compounds would break down in the summer heat and humidity.

However, it *was* a small, family-owned, diversified farm that produced corn, strawberries, cabbages, and a handful of other crops each year. But it was one of a dying breed. All around us, small farmers were disappearing as the farms were acquired by farming corporations. The farm across the street with its measly 150 acres was a relic of the past. The other farms in the area were planting hundreds if not *thousands* of acres at a time; sometimes, swathes of land for as far as one could see out to the horizon were planted in corn.

That farm across the street sold off its land bit by bit. First, one of the back fields was converted into a golf course. Later, additional acreage was sold to housing developers. In the end, the family retained just a few acres—just enough to run a greenhouse-building operation.

I'm no economics expert, but it does seem obvious that when there are lots of small food producers, they are all subjected to the same economic rules. However, it's not hard to imagine what happens if a single producer is able to produce large amounts of food at a low price; in that case, the small producers find themselves unable to compete and they soon go out of business.

Of course, it's easy to spin a conspiracy theory in which big business has set out to undermine the small family farms and the organic ethos all in the name of profit. And sure, the nature of big business is to continue to grow, gobbling up everything smaller. But I suspect that the disappearance of small farms and the erosion of the organic guiding vision are incidental rather than the aim of a grand conspiracy. As we'll see throughout the book, some of these changes are simply a response to growing demand—both for food (with worldwide population continuing to explode) and specifically for *organic* food.

According to the USDA, the demand for certified organic food is continuing to rise. While the U.S. exported more certified organic food than it imported just a handful of years ago, that has now switched as demand for certified organic food in the U.S. now far outpaces domestic production. The USDA reports[1] that in 2013, the value of organic exports was $537 million while the value of organic imports was $1.4 billion. And according to the United Nations, worldwide demand for organic food is higher than production.

Meanwhile, Walmart[2] and other big business interests are seeking to *lower prices* on certified organic foods. In April of 2014, Walmart announced that it will begin selling Wild Oats certified organic food products at stores across the United States at prices *far* below other certified organic products already carried by the stores. In other words, Walmart (and others) may drive down the prices of certified organic foods across the United States. The likely result? Small organic farmers being undercut, unable to compete, going out of business, or, more likely, being gobbled up by big farm corporations.

---

[1] United States Department of Agriculture Economic Research Service (2014, April 14); *Organic Trade.* Retrieved from http://www.ers.usda.gov/topics/natural-resources-environment/organic-agriculture/organic-trade.aspx#.VCskcvldVJk

[2] Walmart (2014). Walmart and Wild Oats Launch Effort to Drive Down Organic Food Prices [Press Release]. Retrieved from http://news.walmart.com/news-archive/2014/04/10/walmart-and-wild-oats-launch-effort-to-drive-down-organic-food-prices

Corporate Control

D rew and Myra Goodman started farming on two and a half acres in 1984. That two and a half acres grew into Earthbound Farms, now a subsidiary of WhiteWave Foods and acquired for $600 million.[3] In a 2009 press release, Earthbound Farms was described as having 30,000 acres of fields, but the 2013 press release described the company as farming 50,000 acres, reflecting a substantial continued growth.

Earthbound Farms isn't the exception. According to the Cornucopia Institute, a non-profit organic advocacy group, 81 independent organic food producers (not farms) existed in the United States in 1995, but now almost all organic food producers are owned by big business.

WhiteWave, the same corporation that acquired Earthbound Farms, has also acquired several other

---

[3] WhiteWave (2013). The WhiteWave Foods Company Announces Agreement to Acquire Earthbound Farm [Press Release]. Retrieved from http://www.whitewave.com/news/north-america/the-whitewave-foods-company-announces-agreement-to-acquire-earthbound-farm

organic and natural food companies, including Silk in 2002 and a full acquisition of Horizon in 2004. WhiteWave itself is a subsidiary of Dean Foods, an even larger food producer.

Other big names in the organic game include General Mills (owns Cascadian Farm and Muir Glen), M&M Mars (owns Seeds of Change), Coca-Cola (owns Odwalla and Honest Tea), Nestle (owns Sweet Leaf Tea), Campbell Soup (owns Plum Organics), Dannon (owns Stonyfield), and J.M. Smucker (owns Santa Cruz Organic and R.W. Knudsen). And just a month prior to this writing, General Mills announced[4] that it will acquire Annie's, the maker of organic and natural bunny-shaped crackers and pasta, for $820 million.

One of the biggest players in organic food is the Hain Celestial Group (owns Spectrum Organics, Arrowhead Mills, Garden of Eatin', Imagine, Walnut Acres, and many others), which reported nearly $1 billion in sales in 2009. Organic Valley, which is also known as CROPP, another one of the largest organic food producers in North America, reported nearly $1 billion in sales in 2013. And some have speculated that the bigger players such as General Mills, Coca-Cola, or Nestle may have their sights set on acquiring large "natural food" companies such as WhiteWave and Hain Celestial.

Some of the big names in natural and organic food have their roots in what would appear to be an authentic

---

[4] General Mills. (2014). General Mills to Acquire Annie's [Press Release]. Retrieved from http://www.generalmills.com/ChannelG/NewsReleases/Library/2014/September/Annies.aspx

commitment to organic principles—local, sustainable, and honest. Stonyfield, the third most popular brand of yogurt in the United States and now owned by Dannon, began in 1983 on a small farm that one of the key early members remembers as "cold and crowded, with a road so perilous that suppliers often refused to come up." The founder, Samuel Kaymen, began the company to feed his children and, in his words, to "escape the dominant culture." Kaymen teamed up with Gary Hirshberg, a man who had previously run an alternative living research center. It would appear that the Stonyfield gang was genuinely an idealistic and ethically pure bunch.

However, in the early 2000s, French giant Group Dannone (also known as Dannon) purchased Stonyfield. At that point, Kaymen left the organization, feeling that the scale of the organization clashed with his personality. Hirshberg remained on as the president and CEO until 2012. During those years, Stonyfield changed considerably because, as Hirshberg put it, his continued employment depended upon "delivering maximum growth and profitability." In order to achieve that growth and profitability, Stonyfield had to make choices that might have felt like "cutting corners" in the old days. Although Stonyfield still sources its fresh milk from North America, it now imports powdered milk from New Zealand, strawberries from China, and apples from Turkey. All of this is done to meet demand with a steady supply *and* increase profitability.

Stonyfield isn't alone, of course. Cascadian Farm has gotten a lot of criticism since its acquisition by General

Mills for adhering to the letter of the law but not the spirit. Like Earthbound Farms, large-scale organic food cultivation from companies like Cascadian Farm or Cal-Organics (a division of Grimmway Farms, the largest carrot producer in the United States) increasingly means farming enormous monoplots. Although they may not be applying banned synthetic pesticides, and although they may rotate crops each year in accordance with organic standards, in most respects, it is difficult to tell these operations apart from their conventional counterparts. A "street view" on Google Earth reveals that the fields of many of these corporations stretch for as far as the eye can see with perfectly uniform crops—in some cases, carrots planted for hundreds of acres and in other cases, such as Earthbound Farms, hundreds of acres of lettuce—all using irrigation systems to support the growth of crops in the desert (as is usually the case). What may have begun as small-scale, ideologically driven, sustainable family farms has become, in many cases, industrial agriculture that is anything but sustainable.

Organic Standards

Many people hold the romantic notion that all foods were produced according to organic standards prior to the middle of the 1900s. However, that isn't strictly true. Toxic substances have been used in agriculture since at least the 1400s when arsenic, mercury, and lead were all used as pesticides. In fact, arsenic-based compounds are reported to have been the most popular pesticides applied in agriculture right up until the 1950s when organochlorines such as DDT became the dominant pesticides. In the 1970s, organophosphates became more popular after organochlorines drew criticism, in large part because of the publication of *Silent Spring*.

What *is* true, however, is that the amount of pesticides used has increased dramatically since the 1950s. Reportedly, pesticide use has increased by 50 fold since the 1950s in the United States. What is it that changed in the 1950s that led to the massive increase in pesticide use? Was it a dramatic change in attitude or values among farmers? Given that farmers have used pesticides for thousands of years and highly toxic pesticides for hundreds of years, it seems unlikely that this is the most reasonable explanation. Another possibility is that manufacturers sought to produce a demand through marketing, and they were successful in doing so. It is likely that this played a part in the increase in pesticide use; there are other factors that most likely played a more significant role.

First, there's population growth; more people means more people to feed. Of course, it can be argued that population growth can be spurred, in part, by increased food availability. But on the other hand, population growth can place a greater demand on food production. In fact, a period starting in the 1940s has been called the Green Revolution because the creation and distribution of agricultural technologies, including synthetic pesticides and chemical fertilizer, is credited with preventing the starvation of nearly a billion people. So at least a part of the increase in pesticide use can be explained by population growth. The United Nations estimates that population growth rates doubled starting in 1920 and then began what appears to be a logarithmic rise around 1950. In 1800 it is estimated that the worldwide human population was one billion, by 1920 it was 1.7 billion, by 1950 it was 2.5 billion, and it has continued to increase up to today with an estimated worldwide human population of 7.2 billion. Increasing pesticide use has (arguably) allowed for significantly greater yields to feed the increasing numbers of humans.

Secondly, there's the increasing industrialization of agriculture. According to the USDA, the number of farms in the United States grew from less than 1.5 million in 1850 to nearly 7 million in 1935. However, since 1935 the numbers have been in rapid decline. In 2012 the USDA Census of Agriculture reported that the number of farms has fallen to 2.11 million. Meanwhile, the number of acres per farm has increased from fewer than 200 in 1935 to 418 in 2012. The *total* amount of land in farms hasn't fluctuated all that much; the same amount of agriculture is being practiced now as in 1935, but it's being done by fewer (but larger) farms.

My sister lives in Kansas, a state in which agricultural interest groups have been conducting a public awareness campaign since the 1970s with billboards informing travelers that "One Kansas farmer feeds ____ people + you." I was visiting my sister last year, and I seem to recall that the signs said that a Kansas farmer feeds 155 people. In 1978, each farmer was feeding 56 people. By 1999, the number was up to 129.[5] The increases are, of course, in part due to increased yields made possible by many of the ongoing Green Revolution technological changes, including chemical fertilizer, synthetic pesticides, irrigation systems, and new generations of high-yield seeds. But the increases are also in no small part because there are fewer "farmers," and each is farming an increasing number of acres.

I put the word "farmer" in quotes because increasingly, farms are not privately owned, family-run affairs as they once were. Instead, an increasing

---

[5] Chartrand, D. (2004, February 14), "One farmer feeds a whole bunch of people," *The Topeka-Capital Journal*. Retrieved from http://cjonline.com/stories/021404/opi_chartrand.shtml

percentage of the farms in the United States and worldwide are big corporations that are answerable to shareholders. What that means is that profit is the number one priority. Although farms that receive organic certification are held to minimum standards, those standards are being manipulated and influenced by the same corporate interests that are heavily involved in organic food production from farm to factory to sales.

In the United States, the first organic certification organization was the California Certified Organic Farmers organization, founded in 1973 amid an increasing interest in organic food. At the same time, the International Federation of Organic Agricultural Movements was founded, the U.S. government banned DDT, and several influential advocates of organic food production published popular books.

However, in 1990, the U.S. congress passed the Organic Food Production Act (OFPA), creating the National Organic Program (NOP) to supersede state-level organic standards and certification. The program is overseen by the USDA, but it is largely informed by a National Organic Standards Board (NOSB), which is an advisory board required by the OFPA. The NOSB is composed of fifteen members, and, according to the OFPA, those fifteen members are to be made of four farmers, three environmentalists, three public interest advocates, two processors, one retailer, one scientist, and one accredited certifying agent.

Obviously, the NOSB is intended to represent a broad range of interests among those with a genuine interest in the principles and ethics of organic food. The members of the board are required to be informed and to make recommendations based upon public interest rather than the interests of individuals or entities (i.e., corporations). However, critics such as Cornucopia Institute argue that many members of the NOSB vote consistently to weaken organic standards in ways that are favorable to the corporate interests they represent.

Among the current members of the NOSB, there are a handful who stand out as suspicious. Two of the four "farmers" are not farmers at all. One of the "farmers" is an organic certifier for Driscolls, which is a berry marketing company that *contracts* with farmers to sell both conventionally and organically grown berries, and, according to Cornucopia, the Driscoll's representative has a measly 17 percent track record of voting in favor of supporting organic standards. Another one of the "farmer" slots is filled by a representative of Organic Valley, a farmer *cooperative* organization, but not a farm. Neither of these two "farmers" are actually farmers unlike the other two farmers, one of whom actually farms 5 acres in Hawaii and the other of whom actually farms 150 acres in Maryland.

Other current board members include representatives from Whole Foods Market, Zirkie Fruit Company, and Earthbound Farms. Past members of the board have been representatives from General Mills, Purepak, Grimmway Farms, Campbell Soup Company, Horizon, Beech-Nut, Smucker's, and Purina Ralcorp. Others, while not actively representing corporate interests during the time of their tenure on the board, have had past associations with various corporate interests that stand to benefit from weakened organic standards. These members have voted alongside (though often in opposition to) genuine environmentalists, conservationists, small organic farmers, and others who vote in ways that consistently represent the public interest rather than corporate interest.

The votes of the NOSB are a matter of public record, and anyone who wishes to can view them. It is interesting to see that their votes are frequently divided with the real small farmers and environmentalists voting one way and the representatives of big corporations voting another way. Take, for example, a vote in 2013 to extend the "sunset" on the allowed use of the antibiotic drug Streptomycin in organic fruit production. Who voted in favor of continuing to use the drug? Representatives from Earthbound, Zirkie, Driscoll's, Whole Foods, and Organic Valley. The vote on continuing to allow tetracycline in organic fruit production was divided along the same lines. As was the vote on the use of genetically modified algae oil in organic food products. As are a great many of the votes on contentious issues.

Interestingly, the NOSB voted *not* to extend the sunset for antibiotic drugs in organic fruit production beyond 2014. Until recently, a two-thirds vote was required to extend a sunset, meaning to extend the duration of an existing allowance within organic standards. However, perhaps in part because contentious allowances such as streptomycin and tetracycline have not been extended, the board changed the rules regarding how sunsets will work in the future.

Previously, votes to allow substances or practices in organic standards automatically fell away (reached their "sunset") after five years *unless* a two thirds majority voted to extend the allowance. However, now the situation has been reversed, and allowances automatically renew unless a two thirds majority votes to *stop* the allowance. The implication is that from now on it will be harder to get an allowance off the standards once it has been approved initially.

Pesticides

Most people are under the impression that organic certification strictly prohibits the use of pesticides in organic agriculture. However, that is not actually true. Instead, organic standards *restrict* the use of pesticides—both which ones can be used and when they can be used. In practice, that amounts to very little pesticide use when compared to conventional agriculture. Also, the list of pesticides that can be used is short when compared to the number of pesticides used in conventional agriculture. According to the U.S. Environmental Protection Agency (EPA), [6] pesticide use in U.S. agriculture was 877 million pounds in 2007, accounting for 63 percent of total pesticide use (industrial/commercial/governmental accounts for 15 percent, and home and garden accounts for 21 percent)

---

[6] Donaldson, D., Kiely, T., Grube A., and Wu, L., Pesticide's industry sales and usage 2006 and 2007 market estimates. US Environmental Protection Agency; Washington (DC): Available from: http://www.epa.gov/opp00001/pestsales/07pestsales/market_estimates2007.pdf

and 78 percent of all conventional pesticide use (meaning substances such as glyphosate and atrazine, produced and used specifically as pesticides). The EPA doesn't report the amount of pesticides used specifically in organic agriculture, but based on the reports of the *types* of pesticides used, it's safe to say that the amounts used in organic agriculture are very small relative to the enormous amounts used in conventional agriculture.

Critics (apparently poorly informed critics) of organic agriculture will often make claims about pesticide use in organic agriculture in an effort to defame the reputation of organic growers. One such claim is that organic growers will often have to apply large amounts of organic-approved pesticides in order to achieve the same results that can be achieved through a small (and therefore less harmful) application of synthetic pesticides. However, the rules of the NOP simply don't allow for the indiscriminate use of pesticides—even those approved for use in organic agriculture. Certified organic growers must have an organic systems plan (OSP) submitted with their certifying agency, and the OSP must include the approved pesticides for use and the conditions under which they may be used. Most pesticides can only be applied after other reasonable steps have been taken to try to remedy a problem. For example, organic growers are encouraged to rotate crops to prevent the likelihood of pest infestations in the first place. Other prophylactic practices are also encouraged. And if an infestation does occur, growers must first take other reasonable measures to reduce the pest population such as using mechanical means (e.g., weeding by hand or removing insects by hand).

There are some exceptions, of course. For example, the application of copper sulfate is allowed once every two years by organic rice farmers to prevent the growth of aquatic pests. Copper sulfate is one of the organic pesticides that is most cited by critics because of the potential harm it can do to the environment as a whole. However, critics often suggest that copper sulfate can be applied indiscriminately, and that is not true according to law. The law allows for very limited use of copper sulfate.

Of course, compliance with the law is another matter entirely, and enforcement by certifying agencies is a variable in the equation. It is certainly possible that some farms may use approved pesticides (or unapproved) for unapproved uses or more frequently or in greater amounts than is allowed legally under organic certification. And it is possible that some certifying agencies may not detect such practices or may look the other way. Certainly, there would be reasons to do so. For example, it really is hard to understand how farms such as Earthbound Farms can plant large monocrops and not abuse the rules. But all the same, as of now, there just doesn't seem to be any evidence that such things are happening on a large scale. Likely it happens on a small scale, of course, as such things usually do. But on a large scale, there isn't reason to suspect that sort of thing yet. So the critics' claims regarding the harmful use of pesticides in organic agriculture (relative to conventional agriculture) are unfounded.

Another common criticism is that certified organic foods have just as many pesticide residues as conventional foods. Or, another variation is to suggest that conventional foods have no pesticide residues. However, neither of these claims is absolutely true, though they do *hint* at some possible truths, as we'll see.

A number of studies have demonstrated that certified organic food often *does* have trace residues of pesticides—often *not* pesticides approved for organic agriculture. For example, a pilot study conducted by the USDA published in 2012[7] found that of 571 samples of organic produce analyzed for 195 pesticide residues, 244 had *some* pesticide residues. However, of those, 121 had levels at less than 0.01 parts per million (ppm), 102 had levels greater than 0.01 ppm but less than the limits of organic certification, and 21 (3.7 percent) had levels greater than allowed by organic rules. Granted, 3.7 percent is significant, but still, let's put this into perspective; the limits allowed by organic rules are less than 5 percent of what is allowed by the EPA for conventional foods. In other words, 3.7 percent of the produce tested in the pilot study had more pesticide residues than 5 percent of the EPA's allowable limit. Do I want to pay organic prices for contaminated produce? No. Do I want to eat synthetic pesticides, even in small amounts? Not really, even though, as we'll see,

---

[7] United States Department of Agriculture Agricultural Marketing Service. (2012, November). 2010 – 2011 Pilot Study Pesticide Residue Testing of Organic Produce. Retrieved from http://www.ams.usda.gov/AMSv1.0/getfile?dDocName=STELPRDC510 1234

minuscule exposure may not produce any harm. But the results of the USDA pilot study are hardly damning and hardly worthy of the criticisms leveled at organic growers when it comes to pesticides.

A UK study published in the British Journal of Nutrition [8] reported that, on average, the level of pesticide residue found in conventional produce is about four times what it is in organic produce. Organic fruits, according the to the UK team, are nearly seven times less contaminated than their conventional counterparts whereas vegetables only a third. The same team also found that organic produce is less likely to contain dangerous levels of cadmium.

The California Department of Pesticide Regulation (CDPR)[9] provides the results of its testing of produce in California for the years 2011 through 2013 on its website. I analyzed the data, and the findings are very similar to what these other studies have reported. In 2013, the CDPR tested over eleven thousand samples for pesticide residues. Of those, only 446 were certified organic. Of those, only 31 had any detected pesticide residues, and only 6 were in excess of allowable limits. On the other hand, nearly half of the conventional samples had pesticide residues.

---

[8] Baranski, et al. (2014), "Higher antioxidant and lower cadmium concentrations and lower incidence of pesticide residues in organically grown crops: a systematic literature review and meta-analyses," *British Journal of Nutrition.* 112(5); 794-811.

[9] You can find the data from the CDPR testing here: http://www.cdpr.ca.gov/docs/enforce/residue/rsmonmnu.htm

Why would organic foods have any pesticide residues? There are a number of reasons. For one thing, in some cases, the detected pesticide is an organic approved substance such as spinosad, which is a product of fermentation of a bacteria. In other cases, residues can be explained by pesticide drift from nearby farms, cross-contamination from processing facilities, or poor handling in markets (many of the samples were taken from grocery stores). Finally, in some rare cases, pesticide residues could be due to dishonest practices on the part of some growers, which may happen more often than we'd like, but probably less often than critics suggest.

All of this discussion, however, leads us to a point which is often overlooked in debates, which is whether or not pesticide residues in foods are actually of concern. If we are to tell the honest truth about the matter, we simply do not know for the simple reason that the relatively short timeframe in which most of the substances used as pesticides have existed precludes any truly long-term studies of the matter. However, as we'll see in the next section, a reasonable guess based on best available information is that pesticide residues on food are *unlikely* to be a serious concern.

Pesticide Residues

Pesticides are toxic—at least, they are toxic to *some* form of life. Not only are they toxic, but they are *fatally* toxic, as indicated by the name, pesti*cide* (-cide is a suffix that means "to kill"). If a pesticide's actions are harmful to humans, then it is obviously sensible to avoid them in significant amounts. For example, the synthetic insecticide chlorpyrifos (which we'll examine shortly) is dangerous for humans as is the organic-approved herbal extract, rotenone, which has been linked with the development of Parkinson's disease among agricultural workers.

However, just because a pesticide is lethal or harmful to *some* forms of life doesn't mean that it is harmful to *all* forms of life. Take, for example, diatomaceous earth (DE), which is a natural silica deposit formed from the cell walls of algae called diatoms. DE is used as an insecticide, but it is mostly harmless for humans and other mammals. Although inhaling large amounts of DE can cause damage to the lungs through mechanical means, *eating* DE is quite safe. In fact, DE is added to livestock feed because it helps to eliminate harmful parasites in the digestive system. Some humans eat DE for the same reason, and reportedly, it may also provide some nutritional benefits, though that point is contentious. The reason why DE is an effective insecticide but harmless to mammals (except when inhaled in large amounts) has to do with its method of action. Insects have waxy exoskeletons. DE absorbs the fats from the exoskeleton, causing the insects to dehydrate. DE also kills some soft-bodied non-insects such as slugs, also causing death by dehydration because the DE absorbs the protective slimy layer. However, mammalian anatomy is different, and the very same effects that cause toxicity in insects and slugs may be beneficial in humans.

At present, the most popular pesticide is an herbicide called glyphosate, better known as Monsanto's Roundup. Based on some studies, Monsanto claims that glyphosate is essentially harmless to humans, is not carcinogenic, and does not accumulate in the body. In the comments section of a Scientific American article[10] regarding a (questionable) study claiming that one of the "inert" ingredients in Roundup is highly toxic, a person claiming to be a Monsanto toxicologist claims that Roundup is, essentially, safer than water. He claims that people who have accidentally or intentionally ingested Roundup suffer few short-term effects and no long-term effects. These claims are in line with the official position

---

[10] Gammon, C., (2009), "Weed-Whacking Herbicide Proves Deadly To Human Cells," *Scientific American*. Retrieved from http://www.scientificamerican.com/article/weed-whacking-herbicide-p/

from Monsanto and a few agencies (such as the California EPA). For those of us who have seen the swathes of brown and gray that remain of dead plants where Roundup has been applied (e.g., along railroad tracks, on guardrails, and so forth), glyphosate may be strongly associated with toxicity. However, that does not mean that it is inherently toxic to humans.

Of course, the supposed lack of toxicity of glyphosate in humans isn't entirely undisputed. Anecdotal reports from others posting in response to the same Scientific American article claim that they have suffered effects from using Roundup according to the instructions and using great precaution. One man claimed that after spraying Roundup on his lawn, he lost motor function in his hand and arm for several hours. Whether or not these anecdotal reports are true, they definitely oppose the stance that Roundup is "safer than water." But I have yet to come across any credible reports of long-term toxicity to humans from incidental exposure to glyphosate in any common Roundup formulation.

Proponents of glyphosate claim that it replaces more-toxic pesticides, including many natural pesticides. Therefore, they claim that it is environmentally friendly—at least in its application (the production of any industrial product is another matter entirely). While this claim may be offensive to many people, that doesn't mean that it might not be true. Of course Monsanto will want to promote its products as being panaceas, beneficial and safe in every way. And if that turns out not to be true, it wouldn't be the first time that a major corporation has lied about the safety of its products and intentionally suppressed evidence to the contrary. In fact, it wouldn't be the first time that Monsanto has lied about the safety of one of its products (Agent Orange, anyone?). However, we shouldn't let cynicism blind us; it is at least *possible* that glyphosate really is very safe for mammals and most insects—though, let's face it, the claim that it is safer than water is absurd. In the EPA fact sheet on glyphosate,[11] there is mention of studies in which various concentrations of glyphosate exposure resulted in everything from stomach upset to decreased body weight to death—though we can assume that the serious effects were noted only at very high concentrations, and here it is important to note that, despite the absurdity of the "safer than water" claim, water when ingested in sufficient amounts will (and does) kill. Additionally, accidental and incidental (e.g., tiny splashes while mixing) exposure to Roundup on the skin and eyes results in serious irritation. On the other hand, the EPA notes that glyphosate is not known to be carcinogenic and that 99 percent of the chemical exits in urine or feces in a short amount of time. So it may be relatively safe, even if not quite as safe as water. Of course, many of us are not only interested in the acute effects of traces of pesticides on human health, but we are also interested in the effects of these chemicals on the larger environment, including plants, animals, fungi, bacteria, and entire ecosystems. But for now, we're only going to look at acute or chronic effects of pesticide exposure on humans through food.

---

[11] http://www.epa.gov/oppsrrd1/REDs/factsheets/0178fact.pdf

Glyphosate is not the only pesticide in use nor the only one found on produce (or in water, human bodies, etc.). Though glyphosate is, by far, the most popular pesticide in use at present, with 180 million pounds used in 2007 in the U.S. according to the EPA report, the next most common pesticide, atrazine, is still used in large amounts—73 to 78 million pounds in the U.S. in 2007. According to the U.S. EPA, atrazine is an endocrine disruptor in mammals, including humans.[12] The EPA states that atrazine exposure is associated with a long list of conditions, including changes in ovaries, adverse liver effects, hormonal changes, immune impairment, birth defects, and decreased birth weight. The EPA notes that these effects can be caused by atrazine-contaminated water and that atrazine contamination of drinking water in the U.S. is common. Other common herbicides include known or possible carcinogens such as metolachlor and acetochlor, both of which are used in the range of 30 million pounds each year.

Insecticides, though used in much smaller amounts, are of much greater concern when it comes to human health implications. That is because the actions of herbicides are generally against plants, which differ significantly from humans. Insects, however, being animals, are *much* more closely related to humans than are plants, and it turns out that chemicals designed to kill insects (by chemical rather than mechanical means) generally cause significant harm to humans—much more so than herbicides. The insecticide chlorpyrifos is

---

[12] http://www.epa.gov/teach/chem_summ/Atrazine_summary.pdf

the most popular, and it is linked with *persistent* adverse health effects in humans when exposure is significant. However, the EPA claims that the average American consumes 0.009 micrograms of chlorpyrifos per kilogram of body mass each day, which is a tiny fraction of the EPA's maximum level, which is set at 0.3 micrograms per kilogram.[13]

Thus far, it may seem like eating certified organic food is likely a sensible way to reduce personal exposure to potentially harmful pesticides. And that *may* be true. For example, a study from Emory University[14] found that switching from a diet of conventionally produced foods to organically produced foods significantly reduced or eliminated urinary metabolites of organophosphate pesticides (such as chlorpyrifos) after five days. But one has to wonder if the results are actually meaningful. The study included a small sample size and was limited to the Seattle, Washington, area, and if metabolites disappeared after five days, that might merely suggest that the body was already able to metabolize and eliminate the minor pesticide residues. Remember, these participants were likely consuming 0.009 micrograms of chlorpyrifos per kilogram of mass, and the study may only have demonstrated that the body can handle that much without harm.

---

[13] U.S. EPA (2011). Chlorpyrifos Preliminary Human Health Risk Assessment for Registration Review (Report).

[14] Lu, C. et al., (2008), "Dietary Intake and Its Contribution to Longitudinal Organophosphorus Pesticide Exposure in Urban/Suburban Children," *Environmental Health Perspectives* 116 (116): 537–542.

On the other hand, for many people, food does not appear to be the primary source of pesticide exposure. That's because, as the EPA and the U.S. Geological Survey have reported, significant levels of pesticides show up in the air, land, and water in many locations. In fact, the levels of pesticide exposure in the *home* is often far greater than the level found in food. The closer one is to an agricultural area, in many cases, the greater the concentrations of pesticides. For example, chlorpyrifos has been detected in surface water near agricultural areas, [15] and the USGS reports that atrazine is now detected in 40 percent of drinking water in agricultural areas. In other words, it would be interesting to see a study similar to the Emory University study conducted in the middle of Illinois or Iowa. The results might be different.

Many pesticides are toxic to humans when exposure is great enough. However, most of us are able to metabolize and excrete them when we are exposed to them in small enough amounts. Not only that, but some have suggested that pesticides are often *hormetic,* [16] meaning that the effects are dose dependent; while large amounts may be toxic, very small amounts may actually prove beneficial.

The theory of hormesis has been applied to many similar phenomena. For example, small amounts of

---

[15] Starner, K., and Goh, K.S., (2103), "Chlorpyrifos-treated crops in the vicinity of surface water contamination in the San Joaquin Valley, California, USA," *Bulletin of environmental contamination and toxicology,* 91(3); 287-291.

[16] Hayes, D.P., (2007), "Nutritional Hormesis," *European Journal of Clinical Nutrition,* 61; 147–159

oxidative stress produced by (small amounts of) exercise produce health benefits, whereas large amounts of oxidative stress from, say, excessive smoking or injury (or excessive exercise), generally produce negative health effects. Alcohol is another example of a hormetic—the consumption of small amounts is associated with improved health whereas excessive consumption is linked with a long list of health problems. This same phenomenon has also been observed in regard to a great many substances found in plants such as polyphenols, carotenoids, and organosulfur compounds—a matter we'll revisit in just a moment.

Some researchers have suggested that we regularly consume *vastly* more (approximately 10,000 times more) naturally occurring pesticides than we do synthetic pesticides.[17] Furthermore, it is suggested that naturally occurring pesticides are *just as toxic* as synthetic pesticides. Naturally occurring pesticides are substances that plants produce to protect themselves from other plants, insects, bacteria, fungus, or any other potential predator. Some examples of naturally occurring pesticides are isothiocyanantes found in brassicas, limonene found in citrus, catechol found in coffee, and caffeic acid found in *just about everything*. Oh, and you'll remember that I said that we'd address polyphenols, carotenoids, and organosulfur compounds. Those substances all may serve as natural pesticides for the plants, algae, fungus, and other organisms that produce

---

[17] Ames, B.N. et al., (1990), "Dietary pesticides (99.99% all natural),".Proceedings of the National Academy of Sciences, 87; 7777-7781.

them. In fact, isothiocyanates, mentioned in the list just a moment ago, are examples of organosulfur compounds that are pesticides, and synthetic allyl isothiocyanates are produced as pesticide products for use in agriculture.

Some examples of polyphenols that act as pesticides include resveratrol, quercetin, and curcumin—all popular nutritional supplements. Resveratrol, for example, is a potent anti-inflammatory substance found in many plants, including significant concentrations in red grapes and in the traditional Chinese herb, known in English as Japanese knotweed. Yet, resveratrol is now being marketed not only as a dietary supplement but also as an agricultural pesticide. Quercetin, a substance found in a large number of common fruits and vegetables, is marketed as an anti-inflammatory supplement and has studies demonstrating its efficacy in addressing a variety of health concerns. It has also been shown to be effective as an insecticide.[18] And curcumin is known to be antimicrobial and insecticidal.[19]

That many plant chemicals could be both pesticidal *and* beneficial for human health shouldn't be surprising. After all, some of the ways in which plant chemicals benefit human health is by *suppressing* immune function (generally in a selective way by reducing chronic inflammation) or by provoking an immune response. In

---

[18] Golawska, S., (2013), "Are naringenin and quercetin useful chemicals in pest management?" *Journal of Pest Science*, 87(1); 173-180.

[19] Griffee, P., "Organic Production of Medicinal, Aromatic and Dye-yielding Plants (MADPs). With inputs from FRLHT," Retrieved from http://ecoport.org/ep?SearchType=earticleView&earticleId=145

other words, they are actually toxins, but in small amounts, they produce a beneficial hormetic effect; a negative hormetic effect can be seen at larger doses. Therefore, it shouldn't be surprising to find that some of these plant chemicals—the very same that are beneficial in small amounts—can be carcinogenic and produce organ failure in large amounts.[20] For that reason, I predict that the current popular trend of supplementing with (unnaturally) large amounts of plant chemicals such as resveratrol, quercetin, and curcumin will fall out of favor because the undesirable consequences will come to light. Either that or they will be found to be benign *and so will some synthetic pesticides.*

To those of us who have shunned synthetic chemicals and for those who have marched against Monsanto, it may be very difficult to accept, but there seems to be a possibility, even a *probability*, that small amounts of some synthetic pesticides may actually have health benefits for humans in the same way as small amounts of naturally occurring pesticides (such as polyphenols) are beneficial for human health because, in fact, many of them are extremely similar in structure and function. That's tough to swallow, but insignificant amount of Roundup on produce may even provide anti-cancer benefits[21] just like quercetin or resveratrol or

---

[20] Dunnick, J.K. and Hailey, J.R., (1992), "Toxicity and Carcinogenicity Studies of Quercetin, a Natural Component of Foods," *Toxicological Sciences*, 19(3); 423-431; Crowell et al. (2004), "Resveratrol-Associated Renal Toxicity," *Toxicological Sciences*, 82(2); 614-619.

[21] Li et al., (2013), "Glyphosate and AMPA inhibit cancer cell growth through inhibiting intracellular glycine synthesis," *Drug Design, Development, and Therapy*, 24(7): 635-643.

isoflavones in soy or clover or alfalfa! Don't get me
wrong; I'm not likely to start popping Roundup
supplements any time soon, but perhaps the widespread
fear of synthetic pesticide residues on food is mistaken.
Many of us are in a position in which we have no
problem taking synthetic nutritional supplements—
some of which are produced by chemical companies—
and yet, arbitrarily, we reject other synthetic substances
despite the fact that they may prove to be no more or
less harmful than the nutritional supplements.

While I know these statements are likely to be
offensive to many people, it is worth examining how our
beliefs are often arbitrary and inconsistent. The truth is
that many of us would reject *anything* manufactured by
Monsanto, even if it was a nutritional supplement that
helped a lot of people. But we often fail to recognize our
blindness when we buy, for example, reverse osmosis
systems, Styrofoam, or plastics produced by Dow
Chemical, the owner of Dow AgroSciences, one of the
major producers of chlorpyrifos and formerly one of the
major (and eventually the sole) producers of napalm.
From an environmental health perspective, industrial
production of just about anything is destructive. But in
terms of the short-term health effects on humans in
terms of residues of food, tiny amounts of Roundup or
atrazine may be no worse than, say, an occasional
aspirin. We don't know that for certain, of course, but
it's not all that far-fetched.

Yes, like any toxic substance, ingesting large amounts
of synthetic pesticides is probably bad for your health.
But here it's good to remember that limits exist for how

much of synthetic pesticides are allowed on food. Various agencies such as the California Department of Pesticide Regulation test food all the time to ensure that the pesticide residues are below the limits. You'll recall from earlier that a number of studies and the CDPR's own numbers reveal that organically grown foods generally contain significantly fewer pesticide residues than their conventional counterparts. However, *the levels found on conventionally produced foods are* already *extremely low.* How low? Well, in general, the limits are described in units of parts per *million* (ppm). For example, the U.S. EPA states that the limit (called a tolerance) for the (actually quite) toxic chlorpyrifos on broccoli is 1 ppm, which means that one part of chlorpyrifos is allowed for every million parts broccoli. That's a lot of broccoli and not much chlorpyrifos. But when it comes to how much chlorpyrifos is actually detected on broccoli, it would seem that the answer is "not much." In fact, in 2013, CDPR didn't report a single instance in which *any* chlorpyrifos residues were found on broccoli. That, despite the fact that chlorpyrifos is used extensively on broccoli in California agriculture according to the California EPA.

It turns out that broccoli is one of the foods that generally has the fewest pesticide residues, but even those foods that are reported to be the worst offenders (the so-called "dirty dozen") still contain very low levels of pesticides according to CDPR data. For example, grapes, reported to be among the most contaminated, did pretty well in 2013 according to CDPR. Out of the 400 test results for grapes listed in the data, 110 had *zero* detected pesticide residues. Of the remaining tests, not a single one exceeded EPA tolerances, and many of them were at least a whole order of magnitude lower than the tolerances. For example, a sample from September 3, 2013 tested positive for residues of cyprodinil, a fungicide that the EPA reports as being of relatively low toxicity. The EPA tolerance is set to 3 ppm while the CDPR test found the level to be 0.254 ppm, a full order of magnitude less than the tolerance. Not only that, but very few samples contained more than a single pesticide residue.

Are pesticide residues on food a genuine health concern for most people? No one can say for sure, but as someone who has fastidiously avoided conventionally produced food for a good decade, I'm starting to suspect that they are not. In fact, I suspect that ultimately, the minuscule residues found on food may make no difference at all since it would seem that the main trade off (nutritionally) when it comes to organic versus conventional is that the organic has fewer synthetic pesticides and more natural pesticides while the conventional is the inverse. And, though no one can say for certain, it really may be a wash. In any case, there simply isn't much convincing evidence that the very small differences either way are significant.

To be clear, I am not suggesting that synthetic pesticide use isn't potentially harmful to health—human and non-human. It certainly may be, and we'll explore that in more depth shortly. But when it comes to the health impacts of eating conventional versus organic food, I doubt there's much difference. Again, I have avoided conventionally produced foods for many years, but after a thorough investigation of the available information, I have to concede that the differences between conventional and organic produce seems to be *negligible*.

Thus far, we've looked only at plant foods, not animal foods such as meat, eggs, and dairy. In the next section, we'll examine the residues of synthetic and other undesirable substances in animal foods.

Chemicals in Animal Foods

U narguably, modern, conventional, industrial food production uses a *lot* of chemical inputs, and when it comes to animal foods such as meat, eggs, and dairy, the amount of chemicals used are often considerably greater than in plant foods. That's because, by and large, animals in the industrial food system are fed a great deal of plant foods (grains and beans, for example) that have been produced using chemical inputs; *plus,* animal producers often include a lot of additional chemical inputs in the animals' food or through veterinary practices. For these reasons, it turns out that animal products are a different story than plant foods. The ethical implications of that are one thing, but at present, let's just look at what residues of these chemicals end up in the food.

First of all, let's look at pesticide residues in these foods. I consulted the USDA data as presented by the Pesticide Action Network to get a sense of how much of the pesticides end up in the foods. I first looked at beef (specifically the fat, which is where pesticides tend to accumulate and we can expect the highest value), and what I found is that the majority of contamination is from a chemical called DDE, which is a (very persistent) product of the breakdown of DDT, which has been banned in the United States for 40 years. So it is reasonable to assume that DDE values in beef are likely the same in organic versus conventional beef.

The next most commonly detected pesticide in beef is cyhalothrin, a synthetic pyrethroid insecticide, but the levels detected range from 0.0005 ppm to 0.034 ppm while the EPA tolerance in beef fat is 3 ppm, meaning that the highest levels detected were two orders of magnitude *less* than the tolerance. I looked at most of the rest of the detected pesticides, also noting that most of them were detected in less than one percent of tested meat, and I found similar results—residues were several orders of magnitude less than the EPA tolerances. I also looked at poultry, pork, eggs, and butter, and the results were very much the same.

Just out of curiosity, I also looked at the pesticide residues in water, including municipal water and bottled water, and it turns out that water is generally contaminated with a far greater number of pesticides and at similar amounts found in meat or other animal foods. All in all, poultry and eggs seem to have the lowest contamination rates while ruminants such as cows and dairy products from those ruminants tend to have the highest levels. Why this might be we can only guess. Perhaps it is because cows are often kept in areas where they are exposed to sprayed pesticides, which increases their exposure, whereas chickens are kept in warehouses and are protected from environmental exposure.

Ultimately, and perhaps surprisingly, the actual USDA numbers on pesticide levels found in animal foods reveal that there's not much to be concerned about. The levels are typically very low. Granted, DDT and its derivatives found in foods is concerning, but given what is known about its persistence, it seems unlikely that it is easy to avoid it or its derivatives whether one eats organic or not. Poultry and pork have much lower contamination than does beef, but not so much that it offers a convincing argument for eating chicken instead of beef.

But pesticides are only part of the picture. USDA rules allow for the use of both natural and synthetic growth hormones in cattle and sheep, and many are concerned about this. Note that growth hormones are *not* administered to any other animals, meaning that all pork, poultry, and poultry products (i.e., eggs) are implicitly free of added growth hormones. There are two primary uses of hormones. The first is the use of something called recombinant bovine growth hormone (rBGH also known as rBST), a synthetic clone of the natural growth hormone produced by cows. It is used primarily in dairy cows to increase milk production, and it has been a cause of much controversy.

One of the major causes of concern regarding rBGH is an ethical one. However, when it comes to human health, the primary concern is that milk from cows treated with rBGH contains elevated levels of bovine growth hormone (BGH) and insulin growth factor 1

(IGF-1). Although the initial reports were that BGH is orally inactive and that it is exclusive to cows, later studies showed that it is orally active and that it affects rats. This raised concern that it may also affect humans. Likewise, elevated IGF-1 levels have been linked with cancer, and therefore many are concerned that milk from cows treated with rBGH has higher levels of IGF-1. Whether or not milk from cows treated with rBGH actually raises human IGF-1 levels more than milk from untreated cows is not yet known, but those who wish to play it safe are choosing to avoid milk from rBGH treated cows.

Because of the controversy about rBGH, the demand for milk from untreated cows is high. In fact, several major U.S. retailers and grocery stores sell *only* milk from untreated cows, and a number of major dairy companies have policies of sourcing milk only from untreated cows. As a result, only 17 percent of U.S. dairies use rBGH, and milk from untreated cows is widely available at no additional cost. Milk from untreated cows will be labeled as such, and most of this milk is *not* organic (though organic standards explicitly prohibit the use of rBGH, so organic milk is also free of rBGH).

The other use of hormones is in meat cows and sheep, but not in poultry, pork, or bison. U.S. law permits the administration of natural and artificial steroid hormones (estrogen, progesterone, and testosterone) in order to increase growth rates. These hormones are normally implanted in a slow-release "pellet" in the ear of the animal. At slaughter the ear is removed and discarded, meaning that hormones are delivered to the animal right up until slaughter. The reason why the hormones may be delivered up to slaughter is that regulatory agencies have determined that the amount of hormones that find their way into the meat is trivial. Well, to be completely honest, I'm betting another major reason is that removing the hormone implants at slaughter is convenient and inexpensive relative to the inconvenience and expense of removing the implants *prior* to slaughter.

All USDA certified facilities test meat for drug residues, including synthetic hormones and antibiotic drug residues. Inspectors may choose to inspect animals if they have any reason to suspect a problem, and random tests are also conducted. A first pass test is done using cheap and fast tests. If the cheap tests reveal no indicators of contamination, then the meat is passed for human consumption. Otherwise, more expensive and time-consuming tests are run to determine if any contaminants exist in the meat. Any meat that is found to have synthetic hormone levels in excess of the limits is excluded for use in the human food supply.

Traces of synthetic hormones in meat are required to be *very* low—so low that they should not cause any effects. In fact, the allowable levels are tens if not hundreds of thousands times less than the naturally occurring steroid hormones in the human body. Not only that, but in the recent reports from the Food Safety and Inspection Service, there was not a single reported incidence of detected synthetic hormones. Granted, not *all* animals are tested for hormone levels, and so when it comes to conventional meat, it's impossible to know with absolute certainty that a particular cut of meat—say, the steak on your dinner plate—is free of elevated synthetic hormone levels. But there's essentially no evidence to suggest that significant traces of synthetic hormones are found in any USDA-certified meat. Meaning that, on average, the hormone levels in most USDA-approved meat will be no greater than those found in 100 percent grass fed, certified organic meat.

With all that said, anyone who is concerned has options that do not require additional cost. Hormones may not be given to poultry, pork, or bison according to U.S. law, and therefore those foods should be free of added hormones whether they are organic or not. It is also possible to find beef and lamb that has been raised without added hormones that is *not* organic, meaning that cost increases should be either non-existent or minimal. The USDA has an approved "no hormones" label that can be added to beef for which the producer has provided documentation demonstrating that no hormones were added to the cow.

Finally, there is the matter of other drugs administered to livestock, of which the biggest concern is generally antibiotic drugs. That is because antibiotic drugs are used extensively in conventional meat, dairy, and egg production. In the United States, producers are allowed to administer antibiotic drugs not only to treat disease but also to prevent disease. And, though it is now being discouraged officially, antibiotic drugs are still used to promote growth. In practice, antibiotic drugs are added to the feed or water of most conventionally raised animals. This practice raises a lot of concerns that have to do with the production of drug-resistant organisms, but in terms of the human health effects of consuming (properly cooked) animal foods from animals treated with antibiotics, the question is, are there substantial residues of antibiotic drugs in USDA approved meat? USDA rules require that producers withdraw animals from antibiotic drug administration for designated time periods prior to slaughter or keeping the milk (in the case of dairy animals). Compliance is *pretty good*, but based on the USDA Food Safety and Inspection Service, it's not perfect.

Antibiotic drugs, even in extremely small amounts, can produce severe allergic reactions in some people and may even send some people into anaphylactic shock. For this reason alone, all animal foods are required to contain no detectable antibiotic residues. In fact, when it comes to dairy, each truckload of milk is tested before use. Any animal or batch of milk with detected antibiotic residues is discarded. So all milk—organic or conventional—that is USDA approved should be free of detectable levels of antibiotic residues.

Unfortunately, when it comes to meat, as we've already seen, not every animal is tested, and the USDA reports that compliance with antibiotic withdrawal regulations is not 100 percent. It is approximately 99 percent,[22] which is close but may not be good enough if you're the one that gets the 1 percent steak and you happen to be severely allergic. Obviously, those who are

---

[22] United States Department of Agriculture, Food Safety and Inspection Service. (2014). United States National Residue Program Residue Quarterly Report 3rd Quarter, FY 2014 (Apr-June, 2014).

allergic can experience unpleasant and even potentially (though rarely) life-threatening symptoms. But for everyone else, trace amounts of antibiotic drugs are unlikely to be a problem. Keep in mind that antibiotic drug traces are found just about *everywhere*, including water. Do these residues pose a potential threat to health? It is possible. But are the traces that might be found in 1 percent of conventional meat likely to be the straw the breaks the camel's back? Probably not.

Still, many people might prefer to avoid the 1 percent risk of ingesting traces of antibiotic drugs that exceed USDA tolerances. For those who want some further assurance without breaking the bank, the USDA has an approved label, "no antibiotics," which can be applied to meat for which the producer supplies adequate documentation demonstrating that the animal was raised entirely without the use of antibiotic drugs. These meats are *not* certified organic, but they are guaranteed to be from animals who were never given antibiotics. Because they are not certified organic, the prices are generally much lower than certified organic equivalents.

When it comes to animal foods, it seems that the regulations are likely to be sufficient to safeguard the health of those who eat the foods. Neither compliance with the regulations nor the testing and enforcement of those regulations is 100 percent, but it's not clear that is a problem. Dairy that is certified to be free of rBGH should be safe because each truckload is tested for antibiotic residues. However, when it comes to meat, choosing meat that has been certified as having no added hormones and no antibiotics may be appropriate for those who wish to have greater confidence in the stringent purity of their food. For most, however, it's simply not clear that such stringent purity guarantees are necessary since the residue levels are generally practically non-existent.

Certified organic foods do offer greater confidence, but that doesn't mean they are failsafe. Although certified organic producers are more closely monitored than conventional producers, that doesn't mean that they cannot or do not break the rules, and sometimes get away with it. What most people don't know is that certified organic producers are required by law to administer drugs, including antibiotic drugs, to their animals if it is believed that doing so is the only reasonable way to prevent unnecessary stress. That animal is then no longer allowed to be processed and sold as certified organic. However, antibiotic drugs are used in certified organic production facilities in some cases, and it may be that on occasion they are used in animals that are then sold as certified organic. USDA tests simply cannot catch all violations. So, yes, the chance of certified organic meat being contaminated with antibiotic residues is *significantly* less than with conventional meat. However, the USDA-approved "no antibiotics" label for conventional meat offers as much guarantee as does organic certification, and in most cases it should be less expensive. Consumer Reports published the results of an investigation[23] in which it was found

---

[23] Consumer Reports. (2012). Meat on Drugs. Retrieved from http://www.consumerreports.org/content/dam/cro/news_articles/health/CR%20Meat%20On%20Drugs%20Report%2007-12b.pdf

that in most large grocery stores in the U.S. (Costco, Walmart, etc.) shoppers are able to find meat produced without hormones or antibiotics at prices close to the average price for conventionally produced meat without the "no hormones" or "no antibiotics" labels.

Of course, avoiding pesticides, added hormones, and drugs is not the sole reason that people choose organic. Another reason is because of concern for animal welfare; many choose organic because they believe that doing so ensures that the animals raised for meat, eggs, and dairy are cared for in ethical and humane ways. In the next section, we'll look at this matter and see how organic stacks up.

Animal Welfare

Those of us who eat meat, eggs, and dairy don't have the luxury of imagining ourselves exempt from the concerns of the welfare of animals kept for food. And many of us *are* concerned. Perhaps we've driven past the heartbreaking and stinky (to put it mildly) yet fairly small feedlot outside of Amarillo, Texas, or the 100,000-cow Harris Cattle Ranch feedlot on I-5 between Los Angeles and San Francisco that can be smelled for many miles in each direction. Maybe we've seen or at least heard about the chicken factories housing mind-boggling numbers of birds in close confinement. And so we want to do something about it; we want to "do our part" to improve conditions.

Of course, some turn to veganism in an attempt to distance themselves from the poor ethics of animal care in food production. But others do not. Sometimes the choice to eat an omnivorous diet is made out of necessity because it is discovered that animal foods are necessary to maintain health for many people. Other times the choice is made because it is realized that the potential harm to life and the ethical concerns cannot be averted simply by eschewing meat, eggs, and dairy—that industrial food production, even the production of carrots and broccoli, can produce just as much harm, hardship, and cruelty as can confinement animal feeding operations (CAFOs).

Those who eat meat, eggs, and dairy who want to improve animal welfare may be seduced by the image presented by organic food companies—the image of animals grazing on green pastures that is actually printed on food packaging to entice us to buy. But is it true? Do organic food producers actually provide dramatically improved conditions for animals in the organic food production system?

Unfortunately, an organic certification does not guarantee significant animal welfare. In fact, as we'll see later, organic certification does not even mean that animals are kept in a way that improves land health— one of the original motivations for the organic movement. Although organic standards *do* set standards for animal welfare that exceed the standards in conventional livestock and dairy production, as we'll see, those standards can be and often are abused.

No doubt, many organic farmers genuinely care about the welfare of the animals for whom they care. While there is no confusion about the fact that the animals are being kept to eventually be food, while they are being kept, many farmers and ranchers feel an obligation to care for and respect those animals. I know because I have known some organic farmers who name their animals, brush their animals, and have genuine love for their animals. However, in terms of the total amount of certified organic meat, eggs, and dairy that is produced, those animals that are cared for with that kind of love and respect—in fact, with *any* love or respect— are very few. And, in fact, most of the farmers I have known who treat their animals with that level of respect are not certified organic.

First, let's consider eggs. Organic standards require that the hens are given access to the outdoors, that they are not raised in cages. Unfortunately, as we'll see, these standards are largely left up to the interpretation of the egg producers, and in the case of almost all large egg producers, the interpretation is made to favor profit, not animal welfare. Furthermore, these standards don't even protect birds from practices such as debeaking and forced molting (through starvation), which are common practices in industrial egg production.

In general, industrial egg producers, including certified organic egg producers, raise hens in large warehouses without any *meaningful* outdoor access. True, in conventional egg production, the hens are allowed to be kept in cages for nearly the entirety of their lives—a practice not allowed in organic egg production. However, in organic egg production, the outdoor access law is often little more than a tiny screened-in porch with a concrete floor, sometimes with such limited space and such limited access that, in practical terms, the hens may never see sunlight. And inside the warehouse there are no minimum requirements for space per bird. A vote was taken by the NOP and it was considered to stipulate a minimum of 2 square feet per hen. That may be better than conventional egg production, but let's face it, it's rotten and simply not a genuine attempt to promote animal welfare.

Other practices common in the industrial egg production business include cutting off the end of the hens' beaks—a practice called debeaking—that is intended to prevent the birds from harming one another. The reason this practice exists is because of the extremely constrained space in which the birds spend their lives, giving rise to conflict. Anyone who has kept chickens in a humane environment can tell you that hens won't peck one another to death when they have adequate space. (Roosters, on the other hand, might. But again, that is when too many roosters are kept together.)

Along with debeaking, another practice common in egg production is forced molting. This is a practice in which, at the end of a laying hen's producing age, she is starved to force a molt and then one more round of eggs. This is a practice that is done *solely* for profit and is clearly not in the interest of the welfare of the hens. This practice is allowed in both conventional and organic egg production.

As a final consideration regarding egg production, it is worth noting that almost *all* laying hens in the United States are born in commercial hatcheries. In fact, the hens in organic production as well as conventional production may come from the same hatcheries. This is true not only of large-scale industrial egg production but also small-scale family farms. There *are* some small hatcheries—I know because I've sought them out. However, the overwhelming majority of all hens, including the ones in most people's back yards, are from industrial hatcheries. There are practically *no* animal welfare considerations given at these hatcheries. The hens producing the eggs for hatching are kept in whatever manner the hatchery sees fit, drugs of all kinds are used freely, and in general, there is no reason to believe that kindness or respect is granted to the animals in large hatcheries. There are *no* certified organic hatcheries.

Next, let's look at dairy production. Organic standards require that all animals in organic production are given outdoor access. In the case of cows, a reasonable reading of the regulation is that dairy cows should be allowed to graze on pasture as much as they want when they are not being milked. Most dairy productions milk cows twice a day—once in the morning and once in the evening. And in my experience, on small dairy farms, the cows are brought in to milk twice a day and then allowed to be on pasture otherwise. The cows usually want to be milked because it relieves the stress of full udders (since the calves are separated from the mothers in most operations), though frankly, most small dairy farmers I know still have to lure many of their cows with a bit of grain or some other treat. (Despite what many seem to believe to the contrary, in my experience, cows prefer grain over grass in moderation in the same way as a lot of humans prefer a candy bar to broccoli.)

However, in larger operations, that isn't the case. I worked briefly on a "small," certified organic, family farm genuinely run by a family and a few employees in which the family seemed to genuinely care about the ethics of organic food production. In addition to row crops and chickens, they also produced beef and milk. Their dairy herd in milk at any given time was approximately 40 cows. That's a lot of cows to milk twice a day for a single milker. The milker worked full-time milking those cows. It wasn't long after he'd finish the morning milking before he had to start the evening milking. Needless to say, the dairy herd lived in the milking barn most of the time, as it simply wasn't practically possible to let the cows out and bring them back in to the milking barn twice a day

But most of the organic milk in the United States doesn't come from small farms with milking herds of 40 or fewer cows. Yes, there are a *lot* of small dairy farms, and yes, many dairy cooperatives pool milk from these small farms and sell them under the cooperative label (for example, Organic Valley). However, the biggest players in organic dairy are the likes of Horizon, which operates a 4000 milking cow "farm" in Idaho. The cows may be certified organic, but is the operation humane? Does it truly live up to the minimum animal welfare standards that most consumers expect when buying organic? I think not.

Interestingly, even at a smaller level, it would seem that many organic dairies aren't meeting animal welfare standards. A study conducted by Oregon State University [24] looked at 292 "small dairy farms" in

---

[24] Oregon State University. (2014). Organic and conventional dairies show few differences in cow health and milk [Press Release]. Retrieved from

Oregon, Wisconsin, and New York over five years. Of the farms, 192 were certified organic—nearly two thirds. The results? Only one-fifth of the farms met minimum cleanliness standards for the herd. Only 30 percent met standards for body condition of the cows. Only 26 percent of the organic dairies applied the recommendations for pain relief when dehorning the cows compared to 18 percent of conventional dairies. (In case it isn't clear, removing a cow's horns is done for the benefit of the human handlers, not in the interest of animal welfare.) Only 4 percent of dairies fed calves the recommended amount of colostrum, and yeah, *all* calves are separated from their mothers at birth, often fed milk replacement instead of real milk. Apparently, even on small farms, animal welfare is lacking whether those farms are organic or not.

Next, let's consider animals raised for meat. Does organic certification improve animal welfare? Not necessarily. Like laying hens, poultry raised according to organic certification is guaranteed a modest improvement in conditions relative to conventional production. Conventional poultry standards are extremely poor, and some major poultry producers have been charged with failure to adhere to even those minimal standards. But, let's face it, when people pay for organic, they expect something that is many orders of magnitude better than conventional practices when it comes to not only quality but also animal welfare, and

---

http://extension.oregonstate.edu/news/release/2014/08/organic-and-conventional-dairies-show-few-differences-cow-health-and-milk

industrial organic poultry isn't delivering on that. It may be better, but frankly, it's not good enough.

Interestingly, I worked briefly at a farm that raised certified organic pasture-raised broiler chickens. One might expect that the quality of life of pasture-raised chickens would be leaps and bounds above those raised in warehouses with concrete floors. And, in a sense, their lives were better because at least they had access to grass and insects. However, those chickens were raised in "tractors," which were 8-by-14-foot enclosures about 2 feet tall that were moved along a pasture so the birds could get access to new ground at least once a day. This, of course, is a common practice among many people who keep small flocks of chickens. In fact, I have kept chickens in tractors. And despite the fact that chickens kept in small, moveable enclosures with low overhead isn't exactly what most people think of when they read the words "pasture raised," it's not so bad, at least in theory. However, the bit that I omitted from the story about the organic farm is that they kept *80* chickens in each tractor. Doing the math, that's 1.4 square feet per chicken. Several large feed bowls and water bowls were also included in the tractor, reducing the space per chicken to even less. Many of the chickens didn't even feather out under their wings since they rarely, if ever, had the opportunity to flap their wings or lift them away from their bodies. Did the conditions meet organic certification standards? Yes. Would any reasonable person consider those conditions to be truly humane? I don't believe so. Were they pasture- raised? Yes. But does the actuality of the conditions match the image that comes to mind when imagining what pasture-raised likely means? Probably not.

What about cows? Unfortunately, when it comes to the welfare of cows, organic certification means very little. In practice, beef cows spend the majority of their lives on pasture. That is true whether they are raised according to organic certification or not. One of the things that cows do that makes them so desirable as food is that they convert grass to meat. In other words, for a relatively small financial input, it is possible to produce a lot of meat. It is generally only in the last months of a cow's life that he or she is "finished" on grain. Grain is more expensive than grass, and it is inefficient to feed cows grain early in their lives. However, the "finishing" process is all about fattening cows quickly, and grain is the way to do that. In fact, during the finishing process, cows gain between 2.5 and 4 pounds *per day*.

The finishing process takes place on a feedlot. If you've never seen a feedlot, then let me paint the picture for you. Cows are placed into pens. Some feedlot operators describe the pens as offering adequate space for the cows, and, to be fair, the cows are rarely crowded side by side in the way that other animals (chickens or pigs, for example) are in confinement operations. But they are crowded all the same. According to the National Cattlemen's Beef Association, cows in feedlots are typically given between 125 and 250 square feet per cow. That sounds like a lot, but 125 square feet is 11 feet by 11 feet and most cows measure over 11 feet from nose to tail[25] and close to 3 feet in width. So we're not talking about a lot of space. And that is in what are called *unsurfaced* feedlot pens, which are simply manure on top of mud or dirt. Surfaced pens, on the other hand, which are manure on top of concrete, allow for even *less* space per cow—as little as 45 square feet per cow. Considering that an average cow occupies not much less than 33 square feet, 45 square feet is the bovine equivalent of poultry battery cages.

Believe it or not, most grain-finished cows end up in feedlots whether they are organic or not. The difference is that in conventional feedlot practices, the cows are fed conventionally grown grain, generally with antibiotics, and they are given hormones to increase growth. In organic feedlot practices, the cows are fed organic grain, and they are not given drugs or hormones. But in terms of welfare, there's not much difference.

The bottom line is that while the National Organic Program gives lip service to animal welfare, in practice, there are few differences. There are *some* differences that are generally positive. For example, it is hard to argue that poultry battery cages used in some conventional poultry operations aren't worse than a cage-free environment, even if that environment affords each bird no more than two square feet of space and those birds never or rarely see daylight. But is the difference enough? Are animals in industrial organic food production actually treated with respect or decency? Are

---

[25] Gilbert et al., (1993), "Body dimensions and carcass measurements of cattle selected for post-weaning gain fed two different diets," *Journal of Animal Science*, 71(7): 1688-1698.

they actually cared for by standards that anyone with a heart would consider humane? The answer is obvious. No, they are not.

To be clear, this is not an indictment of all farmers since there are plenty of farmers who genuinely care for their animals, treating them with not only decency and respect, but also love. But organic certification doesn't guarantee that. And, in fact, the ballooning of the demand for organic food and the increasing interests of big business in the organic food market has only served to make organic certification next to meaningless when it comes to animal welfare.

Environmental Impact

The final matter we'll look at is the relative impacts of organic versus conventional food production on the capacity of the planet to continue to support present life forms, including humans. Critics of conventional food production claim that it is unsustainable and harmful to the health of land, air, water, and entire ecosystems. Meanwhile, proponents of organic food production claim that it offers a sustainable alternative. But rather than believing whatever fits best with our sensibilities, let's take a look.

First of all, are the accusations made against conventional food production true? Are current practices truly unsustainable and harmful? Let's consider what is required in order to grow grain and annual vegetables using conventional practices. Assuming that a field is already in cultivation, a farmer using conventional practices requires gas-fueled tractors, seeds produced by a seed company (often a chemical company such as Monsanto, Dow, DuPont, or Syngenta), chemical fertilizer, and pesticides. Rarely are any of these products produced locally. For example, a farmer in Nebraska may use a tractor, tiller, and planter made in Iowa; a harvester from Illinois; seeds and pesticides from Missouri; and fertilizer produced from components collected in Texas, Kansas, and Minnesota. The pesticides and fertilizer are manufactured, at least in part, from petroleum. The equipment manufacture and distribution also requires a great deal of fossil fuel inputs. Plus, the farmer needs gas to fuel the equipment. That's a lot of petroleum, and that petroleum is sourced from all over the world, maybe including Saudi Arabia, Canada, and Venezuela.

The farmer tills the field at least once a year, contributing to erosion, nutrient loss, and water pollution when the chemicals (pesticides and fertilizer) run off into waterways because the soil is vulnerable after tilling. This is, along with animal manure runoff (mostly from CAFOs), a *major* contributor to water ecosystem harm. For example, a "dead zone" the size of the state of Connecticut exists in the Gulf of Mexico where the Mississippi river empties, due to agricultural runoff. Along with erosion and nutrient loss, tilling also destroys important mycelial networks and disturbs the activities of all the living organisms that work together to create healthy ecosystems.

Once the food has been harvested, it is then distributed using trucks or possibly even trains, using more industrial infrastructure, equipment, and fossil fuel. If the food is intended for consumers, then it will make its way, likely through an intermediary distributor, to grocery stores. If it is intended for food products, it will make its way to a processor that will convert the food stuff into a product before that makes its way to grocery stores. And if the food is intended for livestock, it will go to a livestock food processor.

So are the charges true? Does conventional agriculture and food production fail by any reasonable measures at being sustainable? In a word, yes. Short of some fantasy such as Ray Kurzweil's "singularity," it's hard to imagine any way in which such practices could be sustainable.

What about organic? Does that change things much? Unfortunately, it does not—at least not if we're talking about industrial scale organic agriculture. True, organic growers are prohibited from using most synthetic fertilizer and pesticides. However, in the big picture, the differences between conventional and organic industrial agriculture aren't worth writing home about. Organic agriculture is less harmful, but it is harmful all the same. Tractors are still used. Fuel is still used. Fields are still tilled. And ironically, considering that the organic movement has its roots in soil conservation, erosion still happens, nutrients are still lost, and waterways are still polluted. Food distribution still requires the same number of inputs and comes at the same costs. In the big picture, industrial agriculture is industrial agriculture; some is less bad than others, but none of it is good—at least not if we define 'good' as balanced and sustainable. Keep in mind that the Dust Bowl occurred prior to the Green Revolution, in a day and age when farmers couldn't have dreamed of producing the same effects as are commonplace today.

Let's next take a look at industrial meat, egg, and dairy production. As we've already seen, whether we're talking about conventional or organic, the implications for environmental health are very similar. CAFOs of all sorts, whether conventional or organic practices are being used, result in the same high concentrations of manure and urine that typically contribute to water pollution. Due to the nature of CAFOs, feed needs to be brought in, resulting in major costs for environmental health. And while it is true that antibiotic drug use in conventional practices is likely to contribute to the development of drug-resistant organisms and cause other potential environmental problems, again, when comparing organic and conventional practices, it's merely a matter of degree; both are harmful.

Finally, another uncomfortable matter that is brought up frequently by critics of organic food production is that when it comes to land use, organic is significantly less efficient than conventional practices. Of course, when we factor in the bigger picture, it's hard to say that organic food production produces *worse* environmental effects compared to conventional. However, the simple fact of the matter seems to be that if *only* organic food production practices were used, a great deal more land would be needed for food production than is currently used.

You may recall from earlier in the book that the USDA reports that the amount of land in agricultural use in the United States since 1935 has remained fairly consistent. However, the amount of food produced has increased dramatically, and the number of humans fed has jumped from 127,000 to over 300,000. (It may be that more food is imported now than was in 1935, of course, but in the balance of things, more food is produced per acre than was prior to the Green Revolution.) Organic food advocates often like to claim that organic food production can rival the efficiency of conventional practices. In fact, the Rodale Institute, an organic advocacy organization, has published the results of a 30-year comparison of conventional versus organic agricultural plots *managed by the organization*. Rodale reported that over time, organic became *more* productive than conventional. That is nice, but it's hardly unbiased, and to date no other studies have concluded the same. In fact, all evidence is that organic production falls *well* below conventional, between 40 and 25 percent less at worst.

The reason that organic yields and efficiency is uncomfortable is not merely because it points to a weakness of the argument in favor of converting all food production to organic. Rather, it is uncomfortable because it points to the fact that human population worldwide has increased so dramatically in the past century that it seems impossible to continue to feed us all for much longer *whether using organic or conventional food production practices*. That is uncomfortable for a number of reasons. For one thing, it calls to mind the eugenics agendas of the last century or the Chinese laws restricting children.

In any case, so long as we are allowed to remain ignorant, we may cling to the notion that organic food production will save us all. But when we take a closer look, it turns out that, at least in terms of environmental impact, organic doesn't make good on its promise.

No Happy Ending

Normally, these sorts of books offer a happy ending with some advice such as, "All you have to do is raise backyard chickens, keep a (grass-fed) cow, and grow corn and spinach, and we can save the day and be super healthy all the time! Yay!" But, let's face it, that kind of advice has worn thin. And, anyway, happily ever after is overrated.

Reality is rarely so neat, tidy, and convenient. And in our case, as we've already seen, there's just no way for all of us to feed ourselves by keeping chickens, growing vegetables using no-till techniques, and generating electricity with wind and bicycles—at least not all 7.2 billion humans (and growing). It's a pipedream fantasy. In reality, there's not enough space for that. I've read the books by the people who claim otherwise, but they're either lying or delusional. (Some people actually subscribe to the notion that the Earth itself is expanding. I guess that is *possible*, but it hardly seems *plausible*.)

What we're left with is an uncomfortable, messy reality. And in that context, it's worth revisiting some of the questions that started out this book. Is conventional food production truly sustainable? It doesn't seem so. Is animal welfare in conventional food production what anyone with a beating heart would consider humane? No. Is organic food production better? Yes, but only marginally when it is done on an industrial scale. And that margin is not enough to make it sustainable nor ethical. And, significantly, is it worth paying for? Furthermore, if we do pay for it, are we really supporting a vision of a better alternative? Or are we merely putting dollars in the coffers of the very same big businesses that run and own the whole food production operation?

Yes, there are the small, local, truly genuine food producers who produce healthful food, treat their animals with respect and kindness, and are good stewards of the land. And yes, you can support them. And yes, some of us may have the luxury of being able to choose to produce some of our own food or hunt or gather some of our own food. However, what may once have been a necessity for humans—sustainable food acquisition—is now a luxury for many people, at least in places like the United States. Ironically, sustainable food is out of the financial reach of most people. It may be possible to hunt, trap, and gather one's food without any financial costs, but ironically, financial considerations (as well as legal considerations) often preclude that; fashioning bows and arrows and processing deer could easily turn into a full-time project, leaving little time to secure shelter and clothing, much less have a social life. ("Yeah, I'd really like to come over for bridge night, but I've got to boil my hide glue and fletch my arrows this weekend.") And, contrary to what most in the paleo-diet-zealot crowd would have you believe, it probably wouldn't make you especially healthy.

So it turns out that food that even begins to approach sustainable is now often only available to those who are wealthy or who are willing to make their food one of the major priorities in their life. "Doing the right thing" by purchasing only 100 percent grass-fed local beef, vine-ripened heirloom certified organic tomatoes from a local no-till farm, and the like costs a lot of money. Those producers are true to the spirit of sustainable (and delicious) food production, and so their prices reflect the actual costs of producing that kind of food in that way ($8 for a dozen eggs from chickens guaranteed to have at least 108 square feet each, for example). But it's out of reach for many.

Rather than turn organic or sustainable food into a new religion (which it has already become), perhaps we'd all be better off humbling ourselves and admitting that it's *just a choice*, and not even necessarily a particularly meaningful choice in the big picture. And instead of imagining that we're doing something important when we buy a certified organic beet and a bunch of kale at our local natural food store, looking down our nose at the family pulling out of the McDonald's drive-thru, we could get over ourselves and realize that in the big picture, it really doesn't matter. Food choices are just food choices, and are often are dictated by income level. Snobbery and judgmentalism aren't very pretty.

The story of organic is a seductive one. We live amidst great insecurity, and we often want to have some sense of control or at least some righteousness. Organic offers us that. Local and organic even more so. Then we get to feel that we are "doing the right thing," making the world a better place. In a sense, that's noble. But what we forget is that there's so much that we do not and cannot know, and our views of the problems and the solutions are always colored by our culture, education, income, social status, and a bunch of other stuff that *blinds us* to the bigger picture. That's why people on different points along a political spectrum can have such dramatically different views on things. If any of us were in the other's shoes, we'd see things exactly as they do.

Organic is a nice story, but it's not the whole truth. If you want to choose organic, then do so. If you don't, don't. If you want to, but you cannot for whatever reason, then don't sweat it because it probably doesn't make any real difference. And if you want to be a rebel who is going to change the world—well, good luck to you, but at least now you have the information to steer clear of being a cliché.

Get My Future Books FREE

If you enjoyed this book (Hey, if you made it this far it couldn't have been that bad), you'll probably enjoy many of my other books about health and wellness. And you can get all my new releases in health and wellness for free by signing up for my mailing list at www.joeylotthealth.com. It's simple, it's free, and it's totally honest and legitimate. Nothing scammy or spammy or anything else like that (i.e. I won't be trying to sell you The 7 Dirty Underground Top Secret Weird Tricks for Rock Hard Abs or Young Living Oils). It's just about free books for those who appreciate my work, because I appreciate YOU. Simple as that.

Connect with Me

I welcome your questions, comments, and feedback of any kind. Please feel free to email me at joeylott@gmail.com. I am now receiving so many emails that I cannot always reply to every email. I do read them all, and I do my best to reply to as many as possible. For the benefit of others, I may choose to publish my response to your email on my blog or in book format. I will maintain your privacy and anonymity if I choose to publish my response.

One Small Favor

My sincere goal in writing is to share something that may be of value to you. And I endeavor to do so while keeping the costs low for readers. The success of my books and my ability to reach other readers who may benefit from my books depends in large part on having lots of thoughtful, honest reviews written about my work. You would do me a great favor if you would please take a moment to generously write a review of this book at Amazon.com. This will only take a few minutes of your time, and you will be helping me a great deal. I sure would appreciate it.

About the Author

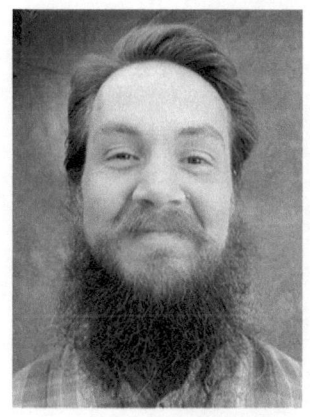

"The secret to happiness is to let go of everything - see through every assumption."

Beginning at a young age Joey Lott experienced intensifying anxiety. For several decades he lived with restrictive eating disorders, obsessions, compulsions, and an inescapable fear. By the time he was 30 years old he was physically sick, emotionally volatile, and mentally obsessed with keeping any and all unwanted thoughts and experiences at bay.

At this time Lott was living on a futon mattress in a tiny cabin in the woods. He was so sick that he could barely move. He was deeply depressed and hopeless. All this despite doing all the "right" things such as years of meditation, yoga, various "perfect" diets, clean air, and pure water.

Just when things were at their most dire, a crack appeared in the conceptual world that had formerly been mistaken for reality. By peering into this crack and underneath all the assumptions that had been unquestioned up to that moment, Lott began a great undoing. The revelation of this undoing is that reality is utterly simple, ever-present, seamless, and indivisible.

Lott's books provide a glimpse into the seamless, simple, and joyous nature of reality, offering a glimpse through the crack in conceptual worlds. Whether writing about the ultimate non-dual nature of reality, eating disorders, stress, disease, or any other subject, he offers the invitation to look at things differently, leaving behind the old, out-grown, painful limitations we have used to bind ourselves in suffering. And then, he welcomes you home to the effortless simplicity of yourself as you are.

Not sure where to begin? Pick up a copy of Lott's most popular book, *You're Trying Too Hard*, which strips away all the concepts that keep us searching for a greater, more spiritual, more peaceful life or self.